MW01171105

Faith & Fitness

The Importance of
Physical Activity
and Fitness
to be a
Healthy & Saved
African American

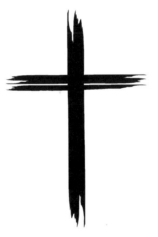

By
Dr. Rev. August Clark Jr., ThD.

Table of Contents

Wise Words from Dr. Lucas Jr.

In today's fast-paced world, maintaining a balanced lifestyle is crucial, not just for our physical well-being, but also for our spiritual and mental health. This truth is particularly relevant for preachers, who often find themselves consumed by the demands of ministry. Dr. August Clark stands out as a beacon of holistic health in this regard. From his days as a professional weightlifter, to his current role as an ordained reverend with a doctorate in theology, Dr. Clark's journey is a testament to the integration of physical strength and spiritual vigor. Dr. Clark's extensive background in weightlifting laid the foundation for his disciplined approach to health and fitness. His transition from the arena of competitive sports to the pulpit did not diminish his passion for maintaining physical fitness. Instead, it enriched his perspective, enabling him to see the profound connection between physical health and spiritual well-being. Earning a theological doctorate further equipped him with the knowledge to address the holistic needs of today's preachers.

The methods outlined in this book have proven successful not just for Dr. Clark, but for many others who have trained under his guidance. Training with Rev. Dr. August Clark has transformed my health journey. My weight dropped from 245 lbs to under 200 lbs, and I gained muscle. The benefits are not only physical but also spiritual. Dr. Clark's teachings instill discipline and sharpen one's spiritual acumen. I highly recommend this book not just for information, but for application. If applied, you'll get the expected results. Scripture underscores the importance of maintaining balance in all aspects of life. As it is written in 3 John 1:2 (NIV), "Dear friend, I pray that you may enjoy good health and that all may go well with you, even as your soul is getting along well." This verse encapsulates the essence of Dr. Clark's philosophy: true health encompasses body, mind, and spirit.

Dr. Clark's dedication and holistic approach to health make him exceptionally qualified to guide preachers towards a healthier lifestyle. His unique blend of expertise in physical fitness and spiritual leadership is a powerful combination, offering preachers the tools they need to thrive in every aspect of their lives. This book is more than a fitness guide; it is a comprehensive manual for achieving optimal health and spiritual well-being.

-Rev. Dr. Larry D. Lucas Jr. Th.D.

My Testimony

Faith & Fitness- The Importance of Physical Activity and Fitness to be a Healthy & Saved African American was a revelational thought given to me after suffering a stroke on March 7, 2018. I spent one week in the hospital. I went through many tests trying to find the underlying reason for the stroke. Doctors could never find the cause. None of the tests were abnormal. I went through physical therapy and made a speedy recovery. I was discharged the following Thursday. I will never forget what this young therapist told me. He said, "Man, most of the time, when people come in the condition you did, they don't normally recover this fast." He continued, "Mr. Clark, whatever you are doing to stay in shape, keep doing it. Your physical condition really helped you tremendously, in strength, to recover so quickly. Plus, you have no neurological dysfunctions." After I saw the effect that it had on my family emotionally, I said to myself, "I have to do all I can to stay alive because I need to take care of my wife and my baby.

I replayed what that young man said to me in physical therapy in my mind, "Good thing you're in shape." A "life-bulb" lit up in my head. Myself, being an African American, who has suffered from an illness that is common amongst people of color, it is important that I warn others about the importance of physical activity and fitness in order to become a healthy person, and an even healthier community. When this idea crossed my mind, my thoughts surpassed weight lifting and jogging. I started thinking about how physical activity and fitness could benefit me in other ways besides just looking good. How could combining these two forces help me counteract some of my everyday life ventures? After personal experiences and a little research, I discovered a few areas of opportunity in my life that could make me even healthier and to become more economical.

Save Money

As aforementioned in my introduction, this revelational thought of being healthy went way past weightlifting in a gym. After seeing so many people in the doctor offices when I was doing my follow-up visits, I was convinced that living a healthy lifestyle can potentially save you money. Yes, physical activity and fitness can lead to healthier spending habits. The old cliches of claiming health as a luxury item no longer holds true. Think of the term health for a moment and write down on paper what the first three things are that you associate your health with. If the first things that come to your mind are gym memberships, plant-based foods, and all sorts of vitamins, then you would be forgiven for thinking that a healthy lifestyle is reserved for the people who are well-off. Although it has been proven that plant-based foods or organic foods do not necessarily have to cost more than conventional food, searching for the right stores to purchase them alone can cost you a lot of valuable time and energy.

One of the first things I decided to do on this quest to healthier eating and saving money was to eliminate some of my expensive habits. The obvious culprit when it came to expensive habits was smoking. I figured that if I could quit for 30 days, I would see myself $4,800 richer in merely a year. Most importantly of all, taking the concerns of my family and friends into consideration as well. I didn't stop there. Those energy drinks and fountain sodas are not only disastrous to the waistline but could also be setting you back over $1,500 a year if it is a daily habit. Factor in the possibility of developing diabetes, which has been linked to fizzy drink consumption, and you will be saving yourself from a future of costly treatments. [1] In an article in the Medical News Today, Markus MacGill wrote a review on "How Soda Impacts Diabetes Risk." In 2016 this review stated that sugar-sweetened beverages contribute to the progression of insulin resistance and prediabetes, the stage before full diabetes. Even though this research finding is not confirmed, it made sense to me. I was diagnosed as being borderline diabetic, so I stopped drinking sodas and drinking more water.

Also, you must challenge yourself to leave the fast food and takeout alone, switching over to mere home cooked meals. For the price of pre-packaged soup that will last you about two days, you can buy the ingredients to make a portion of soup that would last you five days. Not to mention how much money you will save by cutting back on fast food and takeout. By the time a takeout meal gets to your home, a meal could have been cooked and enjoyed, without the double amounts of calories. Process the benefits of cooking your own meals- First, you learn how to cook the foods correctly. Cooking your meals according to a healthy meal plan can significantly improve the way your body processes food. Secondly, your body develops an urge for the intake of food during the cooking phase, digesting them a lot better. You will feel much more fit and more satisfied after meals—once again, this will drastically improve your general quality of life. Save money by cooking your own meals at home. It is healthier and reduces the monthly food bill. You can now better understand how living a healthy lifestyle does more than reduce your waistline.

You will discover other ways that your finances can improve by cutting back on unhealthy habits, pertaining to your own unique lifestyle. Try incorporating the same experiments mentioned in the second and third paragraph half of a year after you have improved your health—my bet is you will be thinking about more affordable things than a gym membership, plant-based or organic produce, and a bunch of vitamins.

Date:

Expensive Habits	Alternative

Tithes:

Bad Foods	Healthy Alternative

To Pay:

○ _____
○ _____
○ _____
○ _____
○ _____
○ _____
○ _____
○ _____

Calorie Maximum	
Calorie Intake	

Water Intake

Proverbs 21:20 NIV

The wise store up choice food and olive oil, but fools gulp theirs down.

10

Date:

_____

_____

_____

_____

_____

_____

_____

_____

_____

_____

_____

_____

Date:

Expensive Habits	Alternative

Tithes:

Bad Foods	Healthy Alternative

To Pay:

○ _____

○ _____

○ _____

○ _____

○ _____

○ _____

○ _____

○ _____

Calorie Maximum	
Calorie Intake	

Water Intake

Proverbs 21:20 NIV

The wise store up choice food and olive oil, but fools gulp theirs down.

12

Date:

_____

_____

_____

_____

_____

_____

_____

_____

_____

_____

_____

_____

Date:

Expensive Habits	Alternative

Tithes:

To Pay:

- ◯ _____
- ◯ _____
- ◯ _____
- ◯ _____
- ◯ _____
- ◯ _____
- ◯ _____
- ◯ _____

Bad Foods	Healthy Alternative

Calorie Maximum	
Calorie Intake	

Water Intake

⬤⬤⬤⬤⬤⬤⬤

Proverbs 21:20 NIV

The wise store up choice food and olive oil, but fools gulp theirs down.

14

Date:

Date:

Expensive Habits	Alternative

Tithes:

To Pay:

○ _____
○ _____
○ _____
○ _____
○ _____
○ _____
○ _____
○ _____

Bad Foods	Healthy Alternative

Calorie Maximum	
Calorie Intake	

Water Intake

Proverbs 21:20 NIV

The wise store up choice food and olive oil, but fools gulp theirs down.

16

Date:

_____

_____

_____

_____

_____

_____

_____

_____

_____

_____

_____

_____

Date:

Expensive Habits	Alternative

Tithes:

Bad Foods	Healthy Alternative

To Pay:

- ○ _____
- ○ _____
- ○ _____
- ○ _____
- ○ _____
- ○ _____
- ○ _____
- ○ _____

Calorie Maximum	
Calorie Intake	

Water Intake

Proverbs 21:20 NIV

The wise store up choice food and olive oil, but fools gulp theirs down.

18

Date:

_____

_____

_____

_____

_____

_____

_____

_____

_____

_____

_____

_____

Date:

Expensive Habits	Alternative

Tithes:

To Pay:

○ _____

○ _____

○ _____

○ _____

○ _____

○ _____

○ _____

○ _____

Bad Foods	Healthy Alternative

Proverbs 21:20 NIV

Calorie Maximum	
Calorie Intake	

The wise store up choice food and olive oil, but fools gulp theirs down.

Water Intake

20

Date:

_____

_____

_____

_____

_____

_____

_____

_____

_____

_____

_____

_____

Date:

Expensive Habits	Alternative

Tithes:

To Pay:

- ○ _____
- ○ _____
- ○ _____
- ○ _____
- ○ _____
- ○ _____
- ○ _____
- ○ _____

Bad Foods	Healthy Alternative

Calorie Maximum	
Calorie Intake	

Water Intake

Proverbs 21:20 NIV

The wise store up choice food and olive oil, but fools gulp theirs down.

22

Date:

_____

_____

_____

_____

_____

_____

_____

_____

_____

_____

_____

_____

Date:

Expensive Habits	Alternative

Tithes:

To Pay:

○ _____

○ _____

○ _____

○ _____

○ _____

○ _____

○ _____

○ _____

Bad Foods	Healthy Alternative

Calorie Maximum	
Calorie Intake	

Water Intake

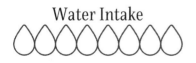

Proverbs 21:20 NIV

The wise store up choice food and olive oil, but fools gulp theirs down.

Date:

Date:

Expensive Habits	Alternative

Tithes:

To Pay:

○ _____
○ _____
○ _____
○ _____
○ _____
○ _____
○ _____
○ _____

Bad Foods	Healthy Alternative

Proverbs 21:20 NIV

The wise store up choice food and olive oil, but fools gulp theirs down.

Calorie Maximum	
Calorie Intake	

Water Intake

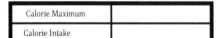

Date:

Date:

Expensive Habits	Alternative

Tithes:

To Pay:

○ _____
○ _____
○ _____
○ _____
○ _____
○ _____
○ _____
○ _____

Bad Foods	Healthy Alternative

Proverbs 21:20 NIV

The wise store up choice food and olive oil, but fools gulp theirs down.

Calorie Maximum	
Calorie Intake	

Water Intake

Date:

_____

_____

_____

_____

_____

_____

_____

_____

_____

_____

_____

_____

Increase Life Expectancy

In my last chapter I talked about how physical activity and fitness can make your budget healthier. Now, I want to inform you that these two can also increase a healthier life expectancy. Let me clarify the fact that these may not add years to your life, but you stand a much better chance at living longer and being healthier than someone who is not physically active or in a fitness program. Numerous studies have shown that regular physical activity increases life expectancy and reduces the risk of premature death. [2] A research on aging from The Journal of Aging Research stated that after 13 studies, it is possible to live 0.4 to 6.9 years longer than someone who is inactive. No, there is not a magic formula that translates hours of physical activity into hours of life gained, but this research suggests that people who are more active tend to be healthier and tend to live longer.

African Americans have the highest rate of mortality in percentage comparisons in Louisiana and possibly America. Hispanics come in a close second place. With the common diseases that plague African Americans such as heart disease, diabetes, high blood pressure, obesity, strokes, and cancer, an inactive person is more likely to succumb to a life of sickness, possibly mortality, in comparison to an active person with the same disease. No one gets to choose their sicknesses of life that could affect our lives forever. However, everyone does get a chance to give it their best physical fight to live longer while dealing with them. There is a great possibility in reducing the fatigue effect and a great chance to beat the disease through daily physical activities. I made a full recovery from a 2018 stroke with no side effects by doing a consistent daily training program. Physical activity is vital to longevity of life.

Date: Time: Weight:

Walking	Running
Minutes:	Minutes:
Distance:	Distance:

Blood Pressure	Heart Rate	Observations

Upcoming
Appointments

_____   _____

_____   _____

_____   _____

_____   _____

1 Timothy 4:8 NIV
For physical training is of some value,
but godliness has value for all things,
holding promise for both the
present life and the life to come.

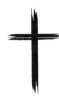

32

Date:

_____

_____

_____

_____

_____

_____

_____

_____

_____

_____

_____

_____

Date: Time: Weight:

Walking	Running
Minutes:	Minutes:
Distance:	Distance:

Blood Pressure	Heart Rate	Observations

Upcoming
Appointments

_____   _____

_____   _____

_____   _____

_____   _____

1 Timothy 4:8 NIV
For physical training is of some value,
but godliness has value for all things,
holding promise for both the
present life and the life to come.

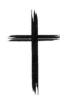

Date:

Date: Time: Weight:

Walking	Running
Minutes:	Minutes:
Distance:	Distance:

Blood Pressure	Heart Rate	Observations

Upcoming Appointments

_____   _____

_____   _____

_____   _____

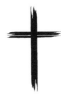

1 Timothy 4:8 NIV
For physical training is of some value,
but godliness has value for all things,
holding promise for both the
present life and the life to come.

Date:

_____

_____

_____

_____

_____

_____

_____

_____

_____

_____

_____

_____

Date: Time: Weight:

Walking	Running
Minutes:	Minutes:
Distance:	Distance:

Blood Pressure	Heart Rate	Observations

Upcoming Appointments

_____   _____

_____   _____

_____   _____

_____   _____

1 Timothy 4:8 NIV
For physical training is of some value,
but godliness has value for all things,
holding promise for both the
present life and the life to come.

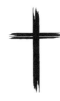

38

Date:

_____

_____

_____

_____

_____

_____

_____

_____

_____

_____

_____

_____

Date: Time: Weight:

Walking	Running
Minutes:	Minutes:
Distance:	Distance:

Blood Pressure	Heart Rate	Observations

Upcoming Appointments

_____   _____

_____   _____

_____   _____

_____   _____

1 Timothy 4:8 NIV
For physical training is of some value,
but godliness has value for all things,
holding promise for both the
present life and the life to come.

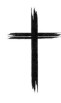

40

Date:

_____

_____

_____

_____

_____

_____

_____

_____

_____

_____

_____

_____

Date: **Time:**   **Weight:**

Walking	Running
Minutes:	Minutes:
Distance:	Distance:

Blood Pressure	Heart Rate	Observations

Upcoming
Appointments

_____   _____

_____   _____

_____   _____

_____   _____

1 Timothy 4:8 NIV
For physical training is of some value,
but godliness has value for all things,
holding promise for both the
present life and the life to come.

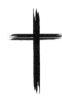

Date:

Date: Time: Weight:

Walking	Running
Minutes:	Minutes:
Distance:	Distance:

Blood Pressure	Heart Rate	Observations

Upcoming
Appointments

_____   _____

_____   _____

_____   _____

_____   _____

1 Timothy 4:8 NIV
For physical training is of some value,
but godliness has value for all things,
holding promise for both the
present life and the life to come.

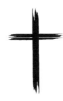

Date:

_____

_____

_____

_____

_____

_____

_____

_____

_____

_____

_____

_____

45

Date:　　　**Time:**　　　**Weight:**

Walking	Running
Minutes:	Minutes:
Distance:	Distance:

Blood Pressure	Heart Rate	Observations

Upcoming Appointments

_____　　_____

_____　　_____

_____　　_____

_____　　_____

1 Timothy 4:8 NIV
For physical training is of some value,
but godliness has value for all things,
holding promise for both the
present life and the life to come.

Date:

_____

_____

_____

_____

_____

_____

_____

_____

_____

_____

_____

_____

Date: Time: Weight:

Walking	Running
Minutes:	Minutes:
Distance:	Distance:

Blood Pressure	Heart Rate	Observations

Upcoming Appointments

_____   _____

_____   _____

_____   _____

_____   _____

1 Timothy 4:8 NIV
For physical training is of some value,
but godliness has value for all things,
holding promise for both the
present life and the life to come.

48

Date:

_____

_____

_____

_____

_____

_____

_____

_____

_____

_____

_____

_____

Date: Time: Weight:

Walking	Running
Minutes:	Minutes:
Distance:	Distance:

Blood Pressure	Heart Rate	Observations

Upcoming
Appointments

_____   _____

_____   _____

_____   _____

_____   _____

1 Timothy 4:8 NIV
For physical training is of some value,
but godliness has value for all things,
holding promise for both the
present life and the life to come.

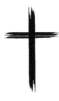

Date:

_____

_____

_____

_____

_____

_____

_____

_____

_____

_____

_____

_____

Reduce the Risk of Injury

Every professional athlete and personal trainer should promote the fact that regular exercise and physical activity can reduce the risk of injury as a person ages. With exercise and physical activities, you are sure to gain increases in muscle strength, bone density, flexibility, and stability. [3] A simple daily fitness program can reduce the risk for and resilience to accidental injuries, especially as you get older. For example, stronger muscles and better balance mean that you are less likely to slip and fall, and stronger bones mean that you are less likely to suffer bone injuries should you take a tumble. It is important to be mindful of physical changes that can increase the risk of common injuries. This includes loss of muscle mass, which results in decreased strength. The loss of elasticity in the tendons and ligaments, which reduces flexibility and range of motion.

Loss of bone mass increases the risk of fractures. Reduced heart, lung, and nervous system function can affect athletic performance. The loss of cartilage results in less cushioning in the joints. Deterioration of balance can increase the risk of accidental falls. We must keep in mind the risk of injury depends on the activity itself and the physical condition of the individual. Your level and frequency of participation also can affect the risk of injury. As an individual ages, it is important that they are sure that they are physically prepared for any chosen activity. Select physical activities and fitness programs that include cardiovascular exercise (running, walking, cycling), strength training, and balance/flexibility exercises. Also remember that cold muscles are prone to injury, so properly warm up and stretch before engaging in any fitness program or physical activities.

Date:

Circle three of the activities below and challenge yourself to do them today.

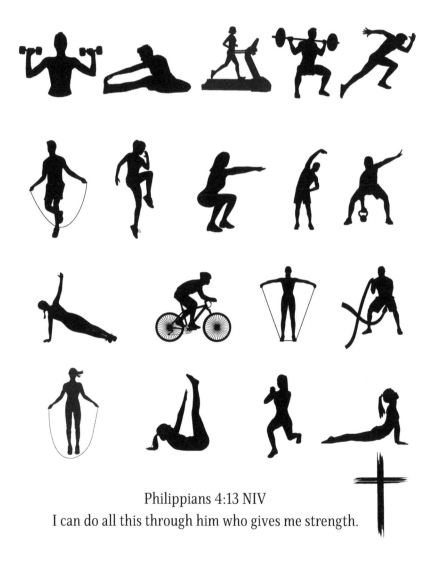

Philippians 4:13 NIV
I can do all this through him who gives me strength.

Date:

_____

_____

_____

_____

_____

_____

_____

_____

_____

_____

_____

_____

Date:

Circle three of the activities below and challenge yourself to do them today.

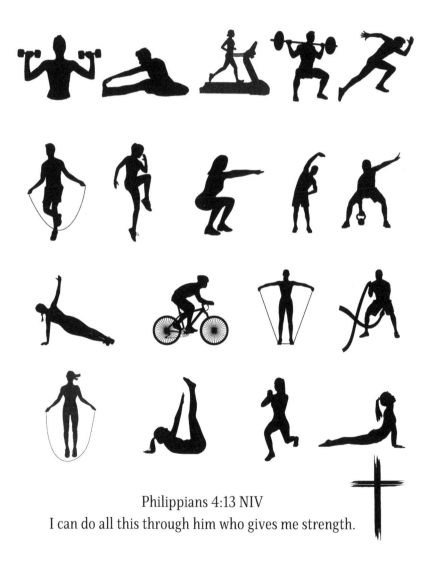

Philippians 4:13 NIV
I can do all this through him who gives me strength.

Date:

_____

_____

_____

_____

_____

_____

_____

_____

_____

_____

_____

Date:

Circle three of the activities below and challenge yourself to do them today.

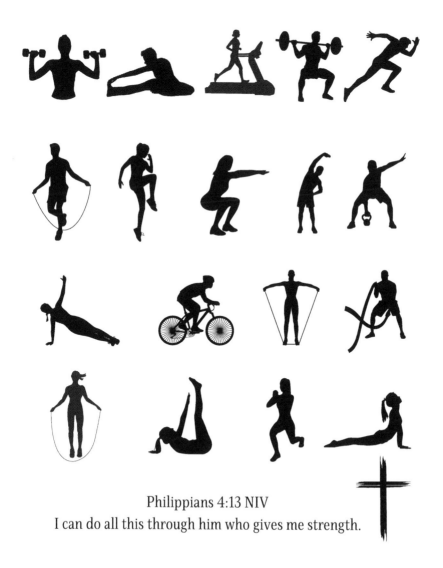

Philippians 4:13 NIV
I can do all this through him who gives me strength.

Date:

_____

_____

_____

_____

_____

_____

_____

_____

_____

_____

_____

_____

Date:

Circle three of the activities below and challenge yourself to do them today.

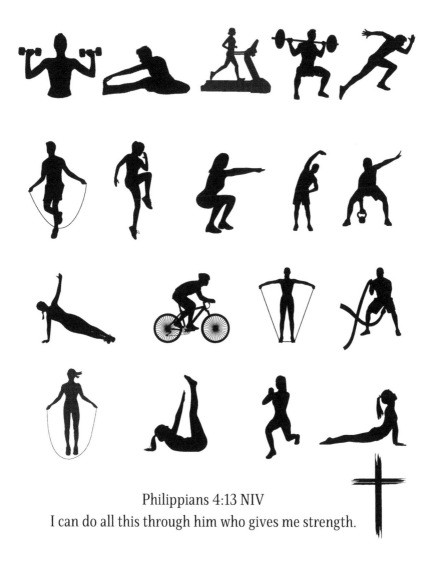

Philippians 4:13 NIV
I can do all this through him who gives me strength.

Date:

Date:

Circle three of the activities below and challenge yourself to do them today.

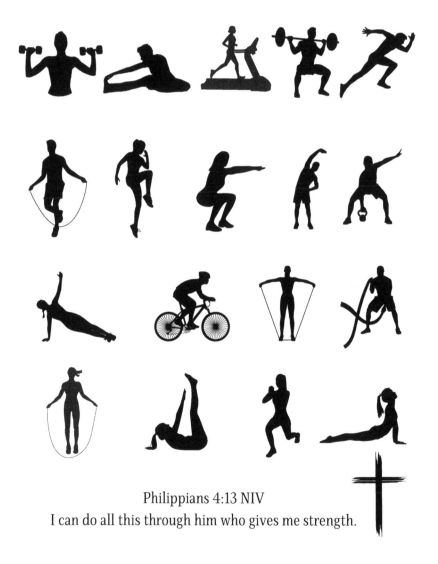

Philippians 4:13 NIV
I can do all this through him who gives me strength.

Date:

_____

_____

_____

_____

_____

_____

_____

_____

_____

_____

_____

_____

Date:

Circle three of the activities below and challenge
yourself to do them today.

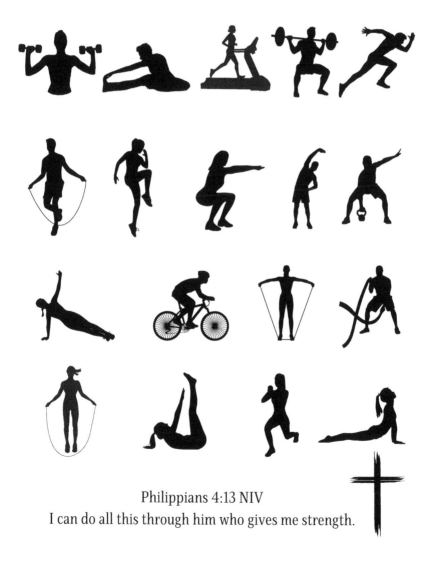

Philippians 4:13 NIV
I can do all this through him who gives me strength.

Date:

_____

_____

_____

_____

_____

_____

_____

_____

_____

_____

_____

_____

Date:

Circle three of the activities below and challenge
yourself to do them today.

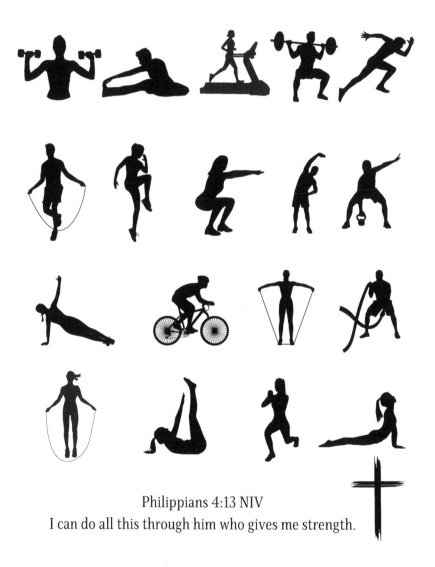

Philippians 4:13 NIV
I can do all this through him who gives me strength.

Date:

67

Date:

Circle three of the activities below and challenge yourself to do them today.

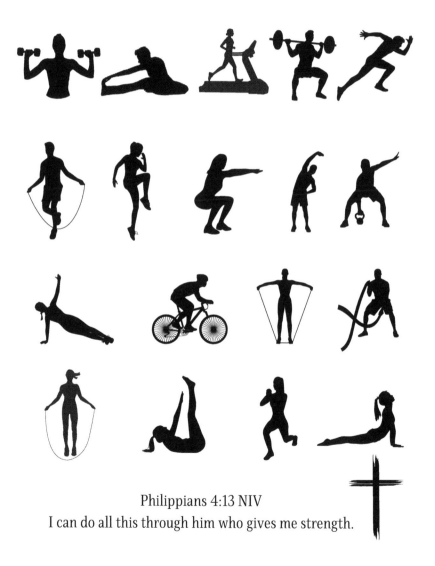

Philippians 4:13 NIV
I can do all this through him who gives me strength.

Date:

Date:

Circle three of the activities below and challenge yourself to do them today.

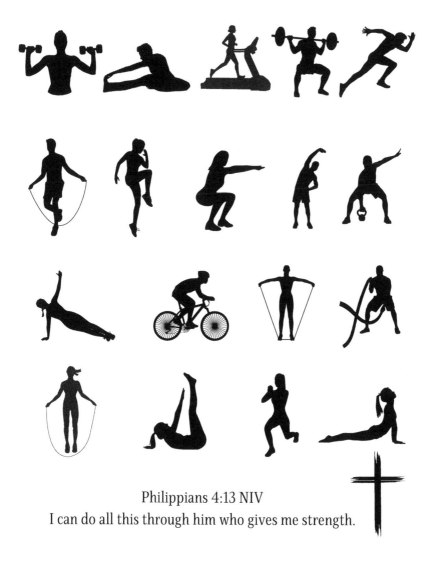

Philippians 4:13 NIV
I can do all this through him who gives me strength.

70

Date:

_____

_____

_____

_____

_____

_____

_____

_____

_____

_____

_____

_____

Date:

Circle three of the activities below and challenge yourself to do them today.

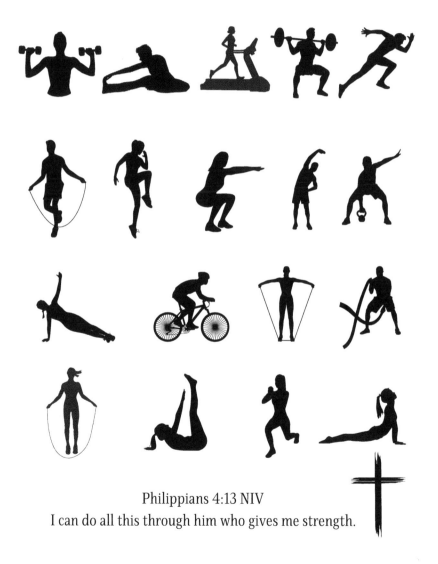

Philippians 4:13 NIV
I can do all this through him who gives me strength.

Date:

_____

_____

_____

_____

_____

_____

_____

_____

_____

_____

_____

_____

Improve Health

Physical activities and fitness programs can improve your health and reduce the risk of developing several diseases like Type 2 diabetes, cancer, and cardiovascular disease. Physical activity and fitness programs can have immediate and long-term health benefits. Most importantly, regular activity can improve your quality of life. A minimum of 30 minutes a day can allow you to enjoy these benefits. There are benefits of regular physical activity. You may reduce your risk of having a heart attack, manage your weight better, lower your blood cholesterol level, lower the risk of Type 2 diabetes and some cancers, lower blood pressure, build stronger bones, muscles and joints, and lower risk of developing osteoporosis. Lowering your risk of falls allows for better recovery periods of hospitalization or bed rest, and you may ultimately feel better. With more energy, a better mood, and feeling more relaxed, you will sleep better.

It has been my experience that physical activity and fitness improves health and also produces a healthier state of mind. A number of studies have found that exercise helps depression. It blocks negative thoughts and distracts you from daily worries. It also provides an opportunity for increased social contact, especially when you are exercising with others. Increased fitness may lift your mood and improve your sleep patterns. [4] Exercise helps stimulate the release of feel-good brain chemicals, such as serotonin, endorphins, and stress hormones.

Date:

How will you use your physical health and well-being to serve others and spread God's love today?

_____

_____

_____

How will you practice self-discipline and self-control in your eating and exercise habits in a way that glorifies God today?

_____

_____

_____

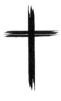

Date:

_____

_____

_____

_____

_____

_____

_____

_____

_____

_____

_____

_____

_____

Date:

How will you trust in God's plan for your fitness
journey and rely on His strength to persevere through
challenges?

_____

_____

_____

How can faith-based practices, such as gratitude and
forgiveness, contribute to mental health and
emotional well-being?

_____

_____

_____

Date:

Date:

What role does nutrition play in maintaining a
healthy body and mind, and how does faith influence
your food choices?

_____

_____

_____

Are there any specific scriptures or teachings that
promote a holistic approach to faith, fitness, and
mental health that you favor?

_____

_____

_____

Date:

Date:

How will you incorporate prayer into your workout routine?

How will you seek balance in your fitness routine and prioritize rest and recovery as a form of self-care and honoring God's design for rest?

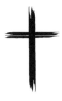

Date:

Date:

How can prayer help alleviate your stress and anxiety?

_____

_____

_____

How can connecting with a community of like-minded individuals through faith-based fitness programs improve your mental health and overall well-being?

_____

_____

_____

Date:

Bibliography

[1] MacGill, Markus. Medical News Today, 2018

[2] Scandinavian Journal of Medicine and Science in Sports. 2009; chapter 19, pp. 419-424

[3] Harvard Health Publishing. 2010-2021

[4] Better Health Channel. Physical Activity is Important. 8-26-2018

Acknowledgements

Thank you to my beloved wife Doretha, my precious baby Makayla, and the cherished memories of my dad August Sr., my mom Ruthie, and my sisters Augustine, Annie Bell, and Audrey. I also extend my gratitude to the Clark/Brent families and Unity Bible College for their support and inspiration.

Love,
Dr. Rev. August Clark Jr., ThD.

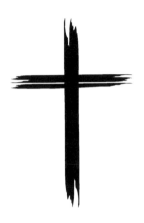

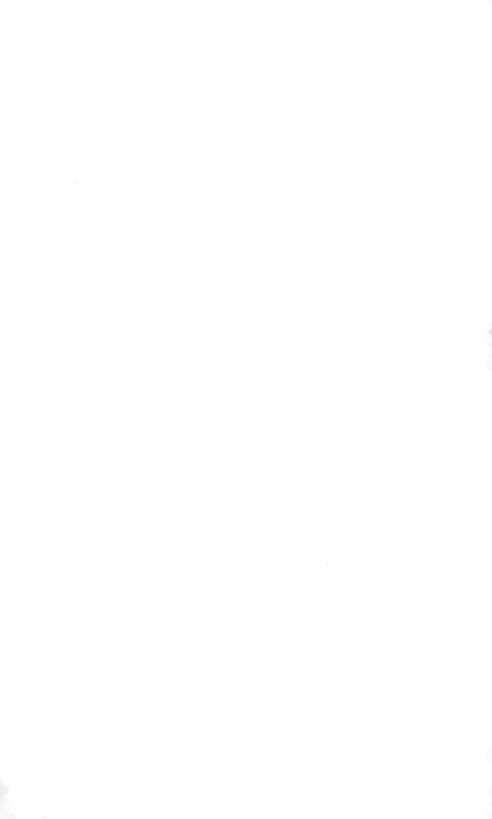

Made in the USA
Columbia, SC
20 August 2024

3e8177e5-14f1-4b82-bdad-8213b894d49bR01